Low-FODMAP Diet

Get Respite from IBS

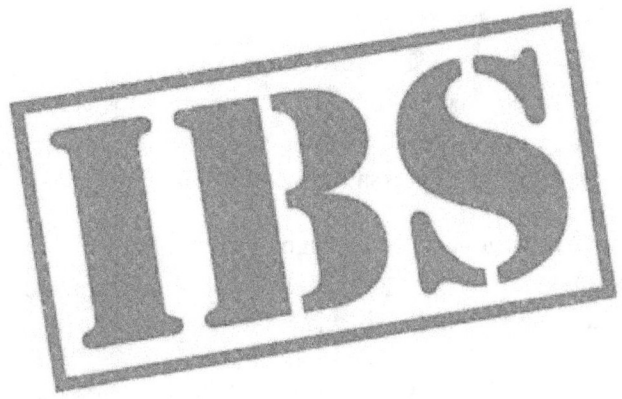

Health Learning Series

M. Usman

Mendon Cottage Books

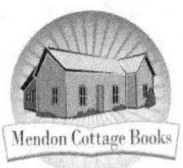

JD-Biz Publishing

Disclaimer

The information is this book is provided for informational purposes only. It is not intended to be used and medical advice or a substitute for proper medical treatment by a qualified health care provider. The information is believed to be accurate as presented based on research by the author.

The contents have not been evaluated by the U.S. Food and Drug Administration or any other Government or Health Organization and the contents in this book are not to be used to treat cure or prevent disease.

The author or publisher is not responsible for the use or safety of any diet, procedure or treatment mentioned in this book. The author or publisher is not responsible for errors or omissions that may exist.

Warning

The Book is for informational purposes only and before taking on any diet, treatment or medical procedure, it is recommended to consult with your primary health care provider.

Our books are available at

1. Amazon.com
2. Barnes and Noble
3. Itunes
4. Kobo
5. Smashwords
6. Google Play Books

Table of Contents

Prelude

If you're reading this book then one thing's for sure: you are either suffering or are in fear of getting IBS/irritable bowel syndrome. I will be getting into the details of the syndrome, as well as, the diet itself later on, but I would first like to tell you that you have certainly chosen the right path against IBS and your money will not go undervalued.

IBS has made people's lives miserable and has devastated their daily routines due to the unpredictable manner of its attacks. Some people have lost all their hopes and have pinned their fate on diets that incorporate artificial drug that only show results in the short term. To address all the prevailing issues related to bowel diseases, the low-FODMAP diet made an entry in the early 2000s, making a profound impact on the whole medical framework. It was swiftly adopted by swathes of people and since then has gained popularity due to its crucial effectiveness. Now it's up to you, as to whether you want to be one of them or not?

I say go for it!

Getting Started

Chapter 1: What is IBS?

Many people are lost on the concept of IBS, let alone FODMAP therefore, there's no point in going straight to the finish line without knowing why you're really running. This book will first explain IBS and conditions relating to it so you would have better knowledge of what you're up against. Following that, FODMAP will be explained in detail.

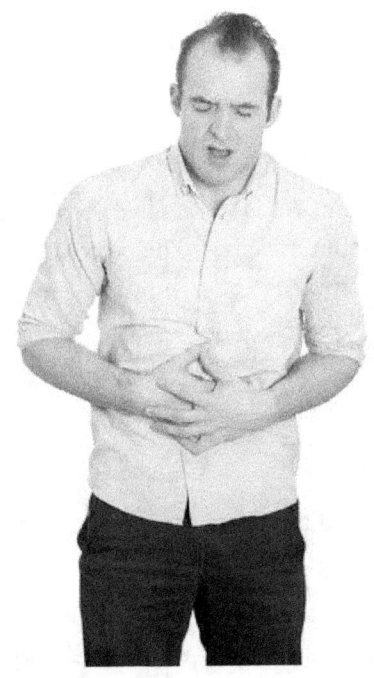

What is IBS or irritable bowel syndrome? Getting right to the point, IBS is a long-term disorder originating in the digestive tract that causes a set of conditions and diseases that devastate one's life. These conditions include, but are not limited to, abdominal pain, mucous in stool, bloating, irregular bowel habits, diarrhea and constipation. The words long-term have not been set in stone and the conditions may decrease in intensity as time passes. It must also be stated that despite all the harshness of the disease, most patients have not yet faced any serious complications that may put their lives in danger, however the fatigue and distress caused by the syndrome is enough to turn one's life upside down.

There are three different ways in which IBS may affect an individual:

1. **IBS with constipation** – the person experiences discomfort, stomach pain, bloating, much delayed bowel movements long with hard stools.

2. **IBS with diarrhea** – the person undergoes discomfort in the form of urgent need to pass stools that are watery.

3. **IBS with a combination of diarrhea & constipation.**

The symptoms of irritable bowel syndrome are largely similar, no matter which type it is. These include:

1. **Pain & discomfort** – this occurs in different parts of the abdominal region which comes and goes. The pain eases with the passing of stool and may sometimes be referred to as a spasm.

2. **Bloating** – swelling of the abdomen which may vary from time to time.

3. **Change in stools:**

i.   Some suffer from diarrhea while some from constipation.

ii. Some people suffer from constipation as well as diarrhea.

iii. Some people form an urgency to pass the stool.

4. **Miscellaneous:**

i.   Nausea

ii. Belching

iii. Headache

iv. Tiredness

v.   Poor appetite

vi.   Backache

vii.   Muscle pains.

viii.   Heartburn

ix.   Irritable bladder

5.   **Anxiety and depression.**

Statistically speaking there are a few factors that aid IBS in developing. People with the most risk of developing IBS include:

1.   **Young adults** – 50% of the recorded cases of IBS involved adults less than 25 years old.

2.   **Gender** – women are more likely to develop IBS than men, 2 times to be exact.

3.   **Family history** – people with a family history of IBS have more chances of IBS taking over.

Chapter 2: Causes & Diagnosis

The causes of IBS are still not known for sure and are a void which is constantly being filled by valuable research from scientists. Still, experts have only been able to chalk down a number of probable causes for the condition that include:

- Environmental factors,

- Dietary factors,

- Lack of proper control from the central nervous system,

- Genetic factors,

- Extra sensitive digestive organs,

- Abnormal response of muscles in the gut,

- Irregularities in the immune system.

Furthermore, evidence suggests that emotional and psychological factors also play a part in the development of irritable bowel syndrome. This statement does not mean that the entire responsibility of this condition can be placed on the nervous system; rather abrupt changes in individual's mood and mental state, like stress and depression, flare up symptoms that lead to IBS.

In some cases, IBS is triggered by certain entities; things that would not affect a normal person. These entities include:

- **Food** – this is one of the most common trigger to IBS. A significant number of patients suffering IBS found their condition getting worse after the intake of foods like milk, alcohol and chocolate; a complete list is given in the subsequent section. Bloating and discomfort was also caused by intake of certain fruits and vegetables.

- **Hormones** – women have found their symptoms to get worse after menstrual periods.

- **Infections** – stomach infections like gastroenteritis are also known to trigger IBS.

A team of researchers have claimed that they have discovered the genetic link in the development of IBS. Scientists from 19 European countries jointly investigated causes of IBS related to genes; 584 cases of IBS and 1,380 control individuals were subjected to tests. The researchers concluded that 2.2% of the IBS patients had a gene mutation that was also found in 1,745 patients of IBS in other areas. They further found out that the gene interrupts with the sodium channel in the gut muscles, which sometimes leads to IBS symptoms.

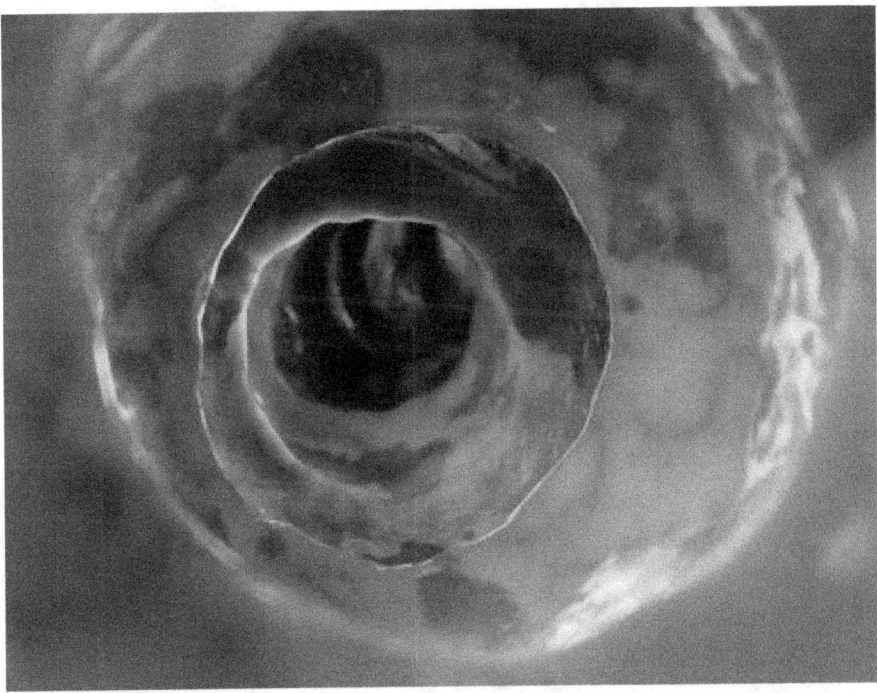

When it comes to testing, IBS has no specific imaging lab that is specialized for the purpose of diagnosing it. Diagnosis of IBS involves a couple of tests and ruling out conditions that produce signs similar to IBS. The following conditions need to be ruled out before any diagnosis is made:

1.   Intestinal bacterial growth,

2.   Celiac disease,

3.   Lactose intolerance.

Most patients are advised to visit their general practitioner for diagnosis, who would recommend a blood test to rule out a couple of conditions. The questions that follow the blood test include:

1.   Have there been any irregularities in bowel habits?

2.   Do you feel bloated more often?

3.   Do you feel any pain in your abdomen?

If there is abdominal pain accompanied by change in bowel habits, the individual most likely has IBS. According to the National Health Service of UK, an individual must have at least two of the following signs in order to be confirmed as an IBS sufferer:

1.   Bloating, hardness and tension in the abdomen.

2.   Need to strain, a sense of urgency to empty one's stomach.

3.   Worsening of symptoms after eating.

4.   Passing of mucus in the rectum.

Patients with more complicated conditions may require further testing; these include sufferers of anemia, swollen rectum and ovarian cancer.

Chapter 3: FODMAP

By this time you may be wondering the meaning of the word FODMAP, right? Well if you are, it must be stated that FODMAP is an acronym for a group of chemicals or carbohydrates that worsen the IBS symptoms.

FODMAP is short for Fermentable Oligosaccharides Disaccharides Monosaccharide and Polyols!

You may not pay much heed to the specifics and to be honest, there is no need to, as long as you know what you're up against. Everything should have started to make sense now, including the title of this book: Low FODMAP diet. The diet that will be discussed rigorously in this book will feature foods that are low in FODMAPs and will help the body regain the strength lost from IBS.

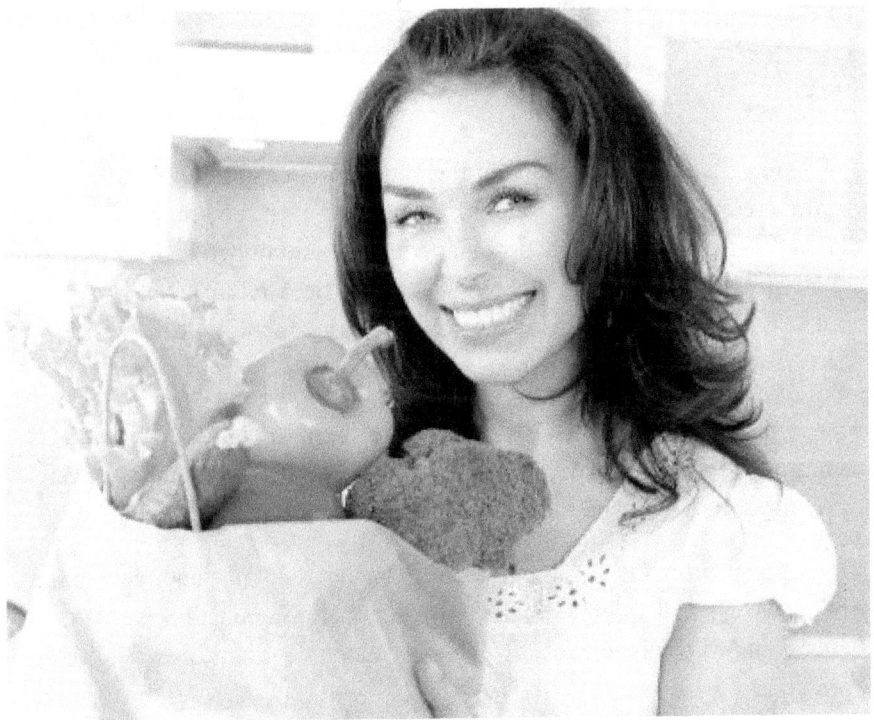

The low FODMAP program is an intensive program which requires a significant amount of discipline to follow. The process of elimination and re-introduction of foods into the digestive system takes about 2 – 6 weeks. The process will start off with cutting out foods that are in included in your diet and are high in FODMAPs; this will be followed by the introduction of foods low in FODMAPs and further reduction in foods rich in the harmful carbohydrates.

A major concern for some people is loss of weight. It must be known that the low FODMAPs diet does not necessarily result in the reduction of weight, especially if you swap out wheat for gluten-free foods. But if you decide to swap out processed foods with fruits and vegetables, you just might be able to see a drop in weight. Research has shown that this particular diet also modifies gut bacteria which play a role in obesity.

FODMAPs are so common in the food we eat that it is almost impossible to avoid them. But with a little care, the intake of these food items can be greatly decreased. The following are a few categories of foods that are rich in FODMAPs:

1.   Fruits:

Fruits may be referred to as one of the biggest sources of FODMAPs. Apples are quite rich in these carbohydrates and even though they have a lot of benefits for the body like supplying vitamins and minerals, they are equally bad for those people who are unable to handle FODMAPs. An apple a day might keep the doctor away for some, but not for those who can't handle these carbohydrates.

Mango might sound like a heartwarming fruit, but for some individuals it can turn their life upside down. The high sugar content of mango can cause difficulties in the gut and interfere with digestive processes.

Watermelon, which is a common thirst quencher, contains enough amounts of FODMAPs to disrupt one's daily life and therefore must be avoided. Other fruits whose intake must be cut down include plums, peaches, cherry, apricot, etc.

2.   Vegetables:

Onion, a well-known vegetable used extensively in dishes because of its ability to add flavor to food, is one of the vegetables that contains FODMAPs. Moreover, leafy vegetables which are considered all so healthy and re-vitalizing are also sources of FODMAPs. You must choose foods according to your capability to digest them; therefore even if you choose healthy foods, you will get no benefit from it but get your digestive system in peril. Other vegetables rich in FODMAPs include beets, asparagus, sprouts, fennel, mushrooms and green beans.

3.   Dairy products:

Dairy products are associated with lactose which is in turn associated with FODMAPs, and the rest as they say is history. Lactose intolerance occurs as a result of intake of food items that rich in FODMAPs and result in bloating and nausea. Milk might be a good source of calcium and minerals but for some it just isn't right.

4.   Spices:

A complete list is given in the following chapter but garlic is the most well-known spice known to cause IBS.

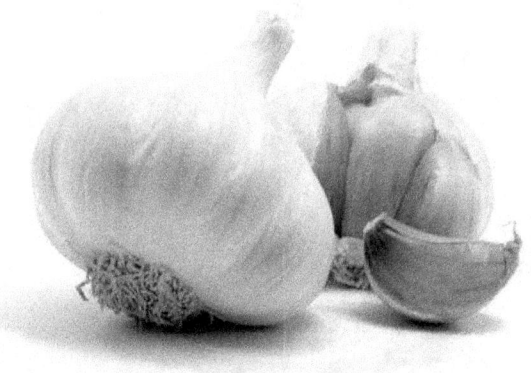

5.   Grains:

Wheat is an essential, staple grain that has been used as a major part of man's diet for centuries. It is used in countless products like porridge, crackers, bread, pies, pancakes, cookies, etc. therefore it would come as a shock to people to find out that wheat also contains FODMAPs. Those who can't handle FODMAPs should avoid wheat at all costs.

Barley, another grain, is also rich in FODMAPs and even though it is an essential part of the morning cereal, it has to be dropped by FODMAP vulnerable individuals.

Chapter 4: Yes or No?

You must be wondering about your daily meal plan after each one of your favorite foods gets taken away from you, right? At first it might seem that FODMAPs are everywhere but if you look in detail, you will find out that there are greater alternatives to the foods that have been declared off the table. Almost every single food item that is allowed or sanctioned for an IBS sufferer has been listed in a categorized way in the following tables:

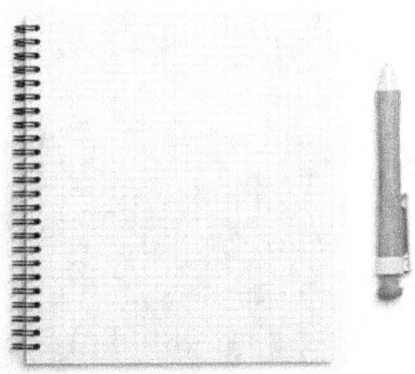

The following is a table that states all the foods that you should avoid when following the low-FODMAP diet:

Vegetables & Legumes
Garlic, Onions, Kidney beans, Leeks, Artichoke, Mango Trout, Asparagus, Mushrooms, Baked beans, Peas, Beetroot, Savoy Cabbage, Black eyed peas, Soy beans, Broad beans, Split beans, Butter beans, Cauliflower, Shallots, Celery

Fruit
Apples, Nectarines, Apricots, Peaches, Avocado, Pears, Blackberries, Persimmon, Cherries, Plums, Currants, Prunes, Dates, Raisins, Grapefruit, Tinned fruit, Lychee, Watermelon, Mangos

Cereals, Breads & Grains

Wheat containing products like breadcrumbs, biscuits, cakes, cashews, egg noodles, regular noodles, pastries, cereals & rolls.

Barley, Bran cereals, Pistachios, Couscous, Semolina, Rye

Sweets, Sweeteners & Spreads

Fructose, Honey, High Fructose Corn Syrup, Milk chocolate, Sugar free sweets, Isomalt, Insulin, Maltitol, Mannitol

Drinks

Beer, Fruit & herbal teas, Dandelion tea, Rum, Orange juice, Sports drinks

Dairy Foods

Cream cheese, Cream, Buttermilk, Custard, Margarine, Ice-cream, Sour-cream, Milk, Yogurt

The following is a table that provides the classes of foods allowed in the low-FODMAP diet:

Vegetables & Legumes

Alfalfa, Ginger, Bean sprouts, Kale, Bok choy, Leek leaves, Broccoli, Lentils, Brussels sprouts, Lettuce, Butternut squash, Okra, Cabbage, Carrots, Olives, Parsnip, Celery, Corn, Parsley, Red Peppers, Courgette, Potato, Pumpkin, Chick peas, Scallions, Chili, Spinach, Chives, Squash, Cucumber, Sweet potato, Eggplant, Tomato, Fennel, Turnip, Green beans, Zucchini, Green pepper

Fruit

Lime, Bananas, Mandarin, Blueberries, Orange, Boysenberry, Passion fruit, Cantaloupe, Papaya, Cranberry, Clementine, Pineapple, Dragon fruit, Raspberry, Grapes, Rhubarb, Honeydew, Strawberry, Kiwifruit, Lemon

Meats, Poultry & Seafood

Chicken, Beef, Pork, Lamb, Turkey, Quorn, Turkey, Canned tuna, Cod, Haddock, Salmon, Plaice, Trout, Lobster, Crab, Shrimp, Mussels

Cereals & Grains

Millet, Wheat free, Bread made of rice, oats, corn, Millet, Oats, Oatcakes, Peanuts, Pecans, Buckwheat noodles, Pine nuts, Rice noodles, Polenta, Porridge, Popcorn, Cornflakes, Potato chips, Rice bran, Pumpkin seeds, Rice Krispies, Quinoa, Almonds, Rice cakes, Amaranth, Rice crackers, Buckwheat, Sesame seeds, Brown rice, Sunflower seeds, Crisp bread, Sorgum, Corncakes, Tortilla chips, Coconut, Walnuts, Hazelnuts, White rice, Macadamia

Sweeteners & Drinks

Pesto sauce, Aspartame, Peanut butter, Barbecue sauce, Saccharine, Chutney, Soy sauce, Fish sauce, Golden syrup, Sucralose, Glucose, Sugar, Jam, Vegemite, Maple syrup, Vinegar, Marmalade, Mustard, Worcestershire sauce, Olive oil, Oyster sauce, Fruit & Herbal tea, Soya milk, Fizzy drinks, Lemonade

Dairy Foods

Butter, Lactose free milk, Lactose free yogurt, Brie cheese, Oat milk, Camembert cheese, Cheddar cheese, Cottage cheese, Parmesan cheese, Feta cheese, Mozzarella cheese, Ricotta cheese, Rice milk, Sorbet, Soy protein, Swiss cheese, Tempeh, Tofu, Eggs, Whipped cream, Gelato

Breakfast

Chapter # 1: Chocolate French toast

Makes: 2-4 servings

Prep time: 20 minutes

Cooking time: 6 minutes

Ingredients:

- 2/3 cup sugar cane juice

- 1/3 cup unsweetened cocoa powder

- ¼ teaspoon salt

- 1/8 teaspoon baking powder

- 4 large eggs

- 1 cup almond milk

- 1 teaspoon vanilla extract

- 8 slices gluten free bread

- ¼ cup butter

Directions:

In a bowl of medium size, whisk all of the dry ingredients i.e. cocoa, sugar, baking powder and salt. Pour in about half of the almond milk and continue to whisk until all the mixture gets a paste-texture and no lumps remain. Whisk in the remaining eggs, vanilla and milk until they become well-blended too. Dip the bread slices into the mixture until the bread turns soggy with the mixture and set aside each slice as it has been dipped. Meanwhile, heat a large non-stick skillet over normal heat and arrange the dipped bread slices on the skillet. Cook for 3-4 minutes, each side and if the bread changes its color too fast, then lower the heat. Transfer the prepared toasts into plates and serve.

Chapter # 2: Burritos

Makes: 4 servings

Prep time: 25 minutes

Cooking time: 15 minutes

Ingredients:

- 1cup chopped green onion

- 1 diced red bell pepper

- ¼ teaspoon red pepper flakes

- ½ pound sausage

- 7 eggs

- 1/3 cup grated cheddar cheese

- 1 teaspoon mustard, dry

- 4 corn tortillas

- ¼ cup FODMAP-free salsa

- ¼ cup FODMAP-free sour cream

- 1 large tomato

- Hot sauce

- Salt & pepper

Directions:

First, heat a non-stick skillet over medium heat and crumble the bulk sausage and cook properly. Remove the sausage, drain off the fat and in the same skillet cook the green onions and peppers until they are charred, which will take about 8 minutes. Add the pepper flakes, pepper, salt and sausage and cook for another 3 minutes. Whisk together the mustard and eggs, followed by the cheese. Add this egg mixture to the skillet, reduce heat to low, and scramble the eggs and cook for 3 minutes. Spread each tortilla with a tablespoon of FODMAP-free sour cream and salsa, then layer with ¼ of the sausage and eggs mixture. Roll the tortillas and top with some diced tomato and cheddar cheese.

Chapter #3: Granola

Makes: 6 servings

Prep time: 20 minutes

Cooking time: 1 hour 15 minutes

Ingredients:

- 3 cups steel cut oats, gluten free

- 1 cup chopped cashews

- 1 cup slivered almonds

- ¾ cup coconut, shredded

- ½ cup caramelized sugar

- ¼ cup raw sugar

- ¼ cup vegetable oil

- ¼ cup FODMAP-free cranberry sauce

- ¾ teaspoon salt

Directions:

First, preheat an oven to 250 degrees Fahrenheit and make the FODMAP-free cranberry sauce. In a large bowl, combine the nuts, oats, raw sugar and coconut and in a separate bowl combine the salt and oil. Combine both the mixtures and set aside. To make the caramelized sugar, heat a 10 inch sauce pan over medium heat. Add ½ cup granulated sugar, a drop of lemon juice and tablespoon of water. Cook with a wooden spoon until the sugar dissolves and the mixture starts to simmer. After the sugar dissolves and the syrup starts to simmer, cook for 10 minutes. Mix the caramelized sugar with the oats mixture and pour onto 2 baking sheets. Cook for an hour and 15 minutes, remove from oven and transfer to a large bowl.

Main Dishes

Chapter # 1: Chicken Rice & Green Bean Casserole

Makes: 6 servings

Prep time: 20 minutes

Cooking time: 50 minutes

Ingredients:

- 10 ounces green beans
- 2 tablespoon fresh chives
- 3 cups diced cooked chicken
- 1 cup celery
- 2 tablespoons olive oil
- 2 cups whole lactose-free milk
- 2 tablespoons coconut flour
- 2 cups white rice
- 1 ½ cup chicken broth
- 1 cup grated gruyere
- ¼ cup grated parmesan cheese
- ½ teaspoon ground pepper
- 1 teaspoon salt
- 1 teaspoon ground allspice

Directions:

Preheat an oven to 350 degrees Fahrenheit. In a large pan, sauté celery along with chives in olive oil until the celery turns tender, which will take about 8 minutes. Push the cooked celery onto one side of the pan without removing the oil from the pan and blend the coconut flour into the oil, cooking for 10 minutes. Slowly add milk to the cooked coconut and blend in the chicken broth until they finely combine together. Simmer liquid mixture for 5 minutes and mix together the spices. Place the rice, gruyere, chicken and green beans in a bowl and toss the spice mixture. Slowly add the cooked liquid to this mixture and pour this combination into a 3 quart casserole dish. Sprinkle the parmesan cheese over the casserole and bake for 25-35 minutes.

Chapter # 2: Beef & Vegetable Stir Fry

Makes: 4 servings

Prep time: 20 minutes

Cooking time: 9 minutes

Ingredients:

- 2 tablespoons fresh ginger

- 1 ½ pounds lean beef

- 2 tablespoons fresh chives

- 1 teaspoon ground pepper

- 6 ounces fresh green beans

- ¼ cup gluten free soy sauce

- ½ cup carrot slices

- 2 tablespoons sesame oil

- 1 tablespoon rice vinegar

- 1 tablespoon sesame seed

- 4-8 Chinese chili peppers

Directions:

Cut the vegetables and meat, grate the ginger, chop the chives and set them aside. Heat the sesame oil in a wok on high heat, add ginger and chives to the oil and stir for 1 minute. Add beef and pepper and continue to stir quickly for 5 minutes. Remove the beef from the pan, keeping the chives and ginger in the pan. Add vegetables to the pan and stir for 2 minutes followed by soy sauce & vinegar. Cover the vegetables, reduce the heat and steam for 10 minutes. Remove the lid, return the beef to the pan, sprinkle with sesame seeds and stir continuously until the meat is warm. Serve it immediately over rice.

Chapter # 3: Chicken & Zucchini Quiche

Makes: 6 servings

Prep time: 45 minutes

Cooking time: 50 minutes

Ingredients:

- 1 teaspoon cumin seeds

- 1 teaspoon sea salt

- 1 teaspoon celery seed

- 2 chicken breasts

- ½ teaspoon red pepper flakes

- ¼ teaspoon ground pepper

- 2 cups lactose-free cheese

- 2 small zucchini

- 4 eggs

- ½ cup lactose free milk

- ¾ teaspoon salt

- ¼ teaspoon ground pepper

- 1 ½ cups grated cheddar cheese

- 1 teaspoon paprika

- 1 FODMAP-free Pie crust

Directions:

First, take the FODMAP-free pie crust and chill it for at least 2 hours; do this ahead of cooking. Preheat an oven to 450 degrees Fahrenheit and in a medium size sauce pan, combine celery, cumin seeds, sea salt, ground pepper and red pepper flakes. Add 2 chicken breasts and cover the pan with cold water. Bring the chicken to a boil, reduce heat and let it simmer for 25 minutes. Remove the chicken from stock and set it aside to cool. Wash the zucchini then slice it into pieces approximately ¼ inch thick and place it on a lined baking sheet. Lightly salt the sheet and bake for 20 minutes, allowing it to cool afterwards. Roll out the FODMAP-free pie crust and place it in a 10 inch quiche pan. Combine cheese, eggs, milk, ¼ teaspoon pepper and paprika in a food processor and pulse several times. Pour the cheese mixture in a large bowl and stir in the chicken. Place a single layer of sliced, baked zucchini on the bottom of the pan and sprinkle ¾ cup cheddar over the zucchini. Pour the cheese/chicken mixture over the cheddar and top in a single layer, with the leftover zucchini. Sprinkle the remaining cheese and bake for 10 minutes at 450. Reduce the heat to 350 and cook for 30 minutes until a golden brown crust is achieved. Allow the quiches to sit in for 10 minutes before cutting and serving.

Chapter # 4: Tacos

Makes: 6 servings

Prep time: 20 minutes

Cooking time: 30 minutes

Ingredients:

- 2 tablespoons chopped chives
- 1 pound ground beef
- 1 can organic tomato sauce
- 1 red bell pepper
- ½ cup water
- Tacos seasoning
- 12 corn tortillas
- 1 tablespoon chili powder
- ¼ teaspoon crushed red pepper flakes
- 1/2 teaspoon paprika
- ¼ teaspoon dried oregano
- 1 ½ teaspoons cumin
- 1 teaspoon pepper
- 1 teaspoon salt

Directions:

Mix together the taco seasonings and put aside. Put a large skillet over medium heat, brown the ground beef with bell pepper and chives and let the fat drain. While the meat is cooking, heat the tortillas in a 350 degree preheated oven for 10 minutes. Stir in the seasonings, tomato sauce along with water; let it simmer for 20 minutes and serve.

Chapter # 5: Polenta Pepperoni Pizza

Makes: 8 servings

Prep time: 20 minutes

Cooking time: 60 minutes

Ingredients:

- 36 ounces precooked polenta

- 2 tablespoons cornstarch

- 3 tablespoons water

- 2 tablespoons gluten free flour

- 1 ½ tablespoon chopped chives

- ½ cup grated Parmesan cheese

- 1 cup grated cheddar cheese

- 2 cups tomato sauce

- 1 tablespoon fennel

- 1 tablespoon chopped chives

- 1 teaspoon salt

- 1 teaspoon sugar

- ½ teaspoon ground pepper

- Pepperoni slices

Directions:

Preheat the oven to 450 degrees Fahrenheit; spray the pizza-pan with non-stick cooking spray. Take the polenta, place in a food processor and process it until it becomes smooth, transferring the processed material into a bowl. Add the water, flour, cornstarch and chives in the food processor and blend them as well. Slowly add the processed polenta and blend it smoothly. Evenly spread the polenta into a pizza pan and bake for 20 minutes; while the crust is baking, make the pizza sauce by taking a medium pan and mixing the tomato sauce, chopped chives, salt, fennel, sugar and pepper. Bring the mixture to boil, reduce heat and let it simmer for 12 minutes. While the sauce is simmering, grate the cheeses and set them aside. Remove the polenta from the oven, spread the sauce on it and top with sliced pepperoni followed by grated cheddar and parmesan cheese. Bake for 25 more minutes, remove from the oven and let it stand for 5 minutes before serving.

Desserts

Chapter # 1: Classic White Cake

Makes: 10 servings

Prep time: 25 minutes

Cooking time: 30 minutes

Ingredients:

- 1 ½ cups sugar

- 12 tablespoons dairy free butter

- 2 teaspoons xanthan gum

- 2 ½ cups all-purpose flour

- 2 teaspoons baking powder

- ¼ teaspoons salt

- ¾ cup whole milk

- 6 large egg whites

- 2 teaspoons vanilla extract

- 3 9-inch round pans

Directions:

Preheat an oven to 350 degrees and spray the sides of a pan with non-stick spray; line the bottom with wax-paper. In a large bowl, beat the sugar and butter for 10 minutes, until it turns light and fluffy. Sift the flour into a large bowl and whisk together the flour, gum, salt and baking powder. Combine the vanilla extract and milk and add half the flour-mixture to butter-mixture and the other half to milk-mixture; repeat until all ingredients are combined. Scrape the bowl and do not over mix. Whip the egg whites until peaks form, fold the egg whites into batter and pour into prepared pans. Bake for 30 minutes or until a fork comes out clean when inserted in its center. Cool the cake for 5 minutes, then remove the paper and let it cool completely before serving.

Chapter # 2: Chocolate Peanut-Butter Bars

Makes: 20 servings

Prep time: 15 minutes

Cooking time: 1 minute

Ingredients:

Chocolate cookie crust

- 1 ½ cups sugar, granulated

- ¾ cup gluten free flour

- ¾ cup unsweetened cocoa powder

- 1 teaspoon xanthan gum

- ¼ teaspoon cinnamon

- 1/8 teaspoon salt

- ½ cups dairy free butter

Peanut Butter Filling

- 1 ¼ cup FODMAP-free peanut butter

- 1 cup lactose-free vanilla creamer

- ½ teaspoon cinnamon

- ½ teaspoon vanilla

- ¼ teaspoon cloves

- ¼ teaspoon nutmeg

- 3 ¼ cups powdered sugar

FODMAP-free Fudge

- ¼ cup unsweetened cocoa powder

- ½ cup dairy-free butter

- 1 ½ cups white sugar, granulated

- 5 tablespoons whole milk

- 1 tablespoons lemon juice

- ½ teaspoon cinnamon

Directions:

Make the Chocolate Cookie Crust and allow it to cool. In order to make the filling, stir together the cloves, cinnamon and nutmeg; put this aside. Using an electric mixer beat the peanut butter until it turns creamy. Add the creamer and vanilla to the peanut butter and mix well followed by addition of spice mixture to peanut butter. Mix in the powdered sugar and stir in chopped peanuts; spread the peanut butter mixture over the Chocolate Cookie Crust and put this in a refrigerator while making the Fudge topping. Spread the topping immediately over the peanut butter and seal it to the edges. Freeze for an hour before serving the bars.

Chapter # 3: Salted Caramel Ice-cream

Makes: 1 quart

Prep time: 30 minutes

Cooking time: 4 minutes

Ingredients:

- 1 ¼ cups divided sugar

- 2 ¼ cups French vanilla Soymilk creamer

- ½ teaspoon clear vanilla extract

- ½ teaspoons flaky sea salt

- 1 cup whole milk

- 4 large eggs

Directions:

First, heat 1 cup of white sugar in a dry 10-inch skillet over medium heat, making sure that the sugar is evenly stirred. When the sugar melts, stop stirring and let it cook until it is dark amber in color. Add 1 ¼ cups of French vanilla creamer and cook by stirring it until all the caramel has dissolved; transfer this to a bowl and stir in the sea salt and vanilla. Cool to room temperature by putting the bowl in a refrigerator while preparing the custard. While the caramel is cooling, bring the lactose-free milk, remaining French soymilk and ¼ cup sugar to a boil in a heavy saucepan. Whisk the eggs in a bowl; add half of the hot milk in a slow stream, whisking the mixture constantly as you do so. Pour the egg/milk mixture into the remaining sauce in the pan and cook with a wooden spoon until the custard coats the spoon, at about 170 degrees Fahrenheit. Pour the custard through a sieve into a bowl and stir in the cooled caramel. Cover the finished mixture with a plastic wrap and seal the edges. Chill custard for 3 to 6 hours after which pour it into an ice-cream maker, blending it for 20 minutes. Put the ice cream in the freezer so it can firm up.

Conclusion

By now you have gotten the true essence of the Low-FODMAP diet and the mechanisms by which it relives you from IBS discomfort. The book starts off from the basics and assumes that you have no prior knowledge of the disease and ends up with telling its cures through the intake of low FODMAP diet. All the related material has been provided in detail so no doubt will be left in your mind about the effectiveness of this diet. Recipes for breakfast, entrees as well as desserts have been given to ease the transition. The concept is simple which is explained by the name of the diet itself; by limiting the intake of harmful compounds, you may prevent the onset of discomfort and unwanted nausea.

Follow the diet; stay happy & best of luck!

References

http://www.123rf.com/photo_26101405_ibs-irritable-bowel-syndrome-red-rubber-stamp-over-a-white-background.html?term=ibs

http://www.123rf.com/photo_18451714_inside-of-an-unhealthy-colon.html?term=bowel%20syndrome

http://www.123rf.com/photo_26104759_closeup-portrait-of-miserable-upset-young-man-doubling-over-in-acute-body-stomach-pain-looking-very-.html?term=bowel%20syndrome

http://www.123rf.com/photo_18941095_happy-young-woman-with-vegetables-in-shopping-bag-diet-concept.html?term=diet

http://fotolia.com/id/37202640

http://fotolia.com/id/52133132

Author Bio

Muhammad Usman is a distinguished medical graduate of Allama Iqbal medical college (AIMC). He is a professional writer who has been in the field for more than 4 years. During this time he has produced 10,000+ articles, blogs and eBooks on various niches related to diseases, health, fitness, nutrition and well-being. He is a regular contributor to several journals related to medicine and surgery. He is the editor of several journals and newspapers.

Check out some of the other JD-Biz Publishing books

Gardening Series on Amazon

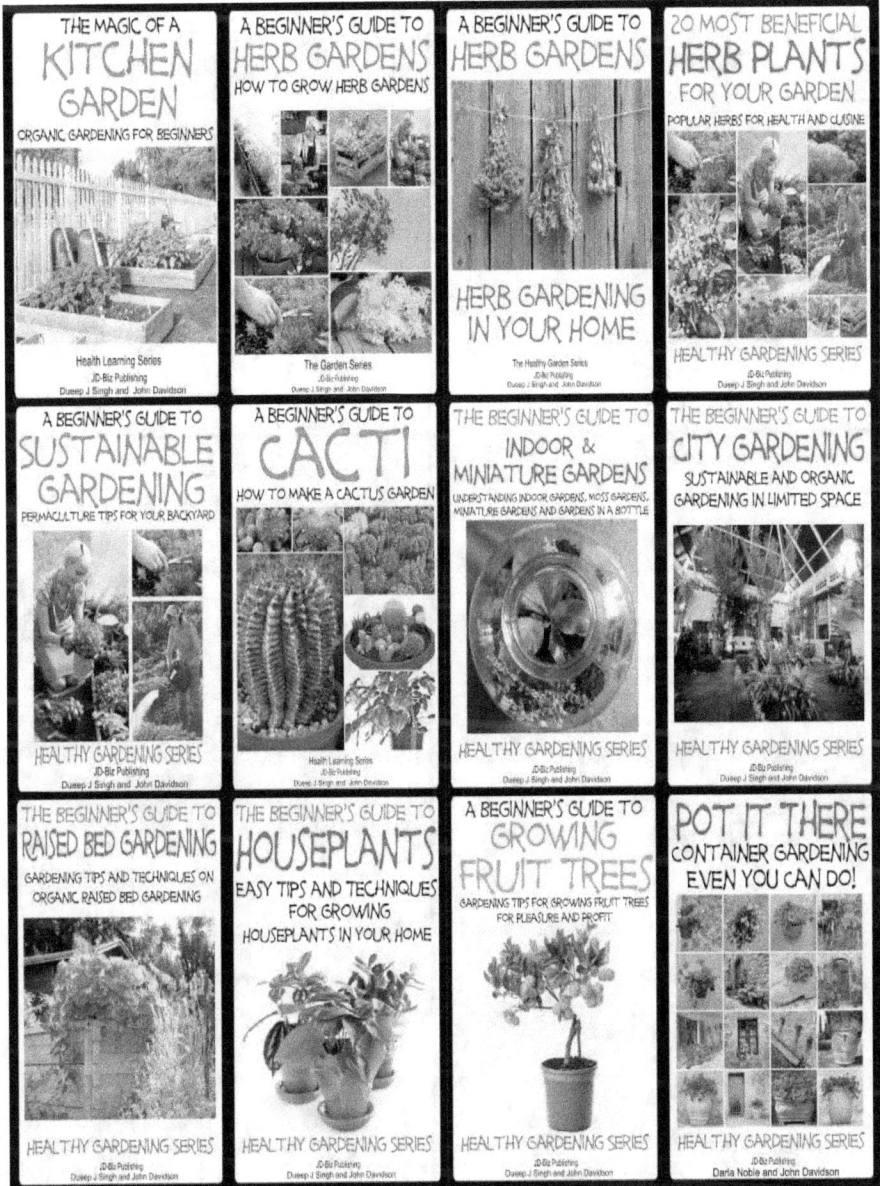

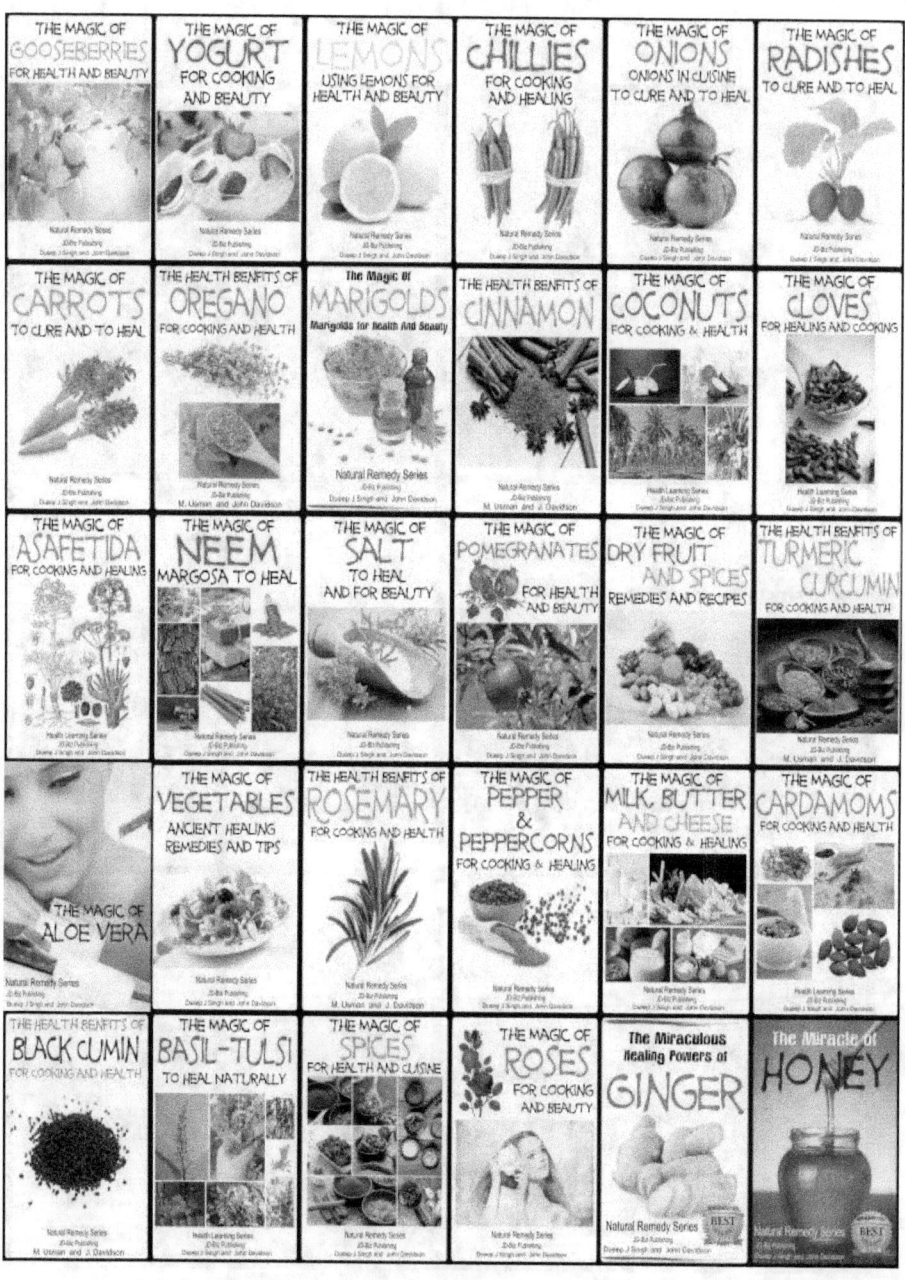

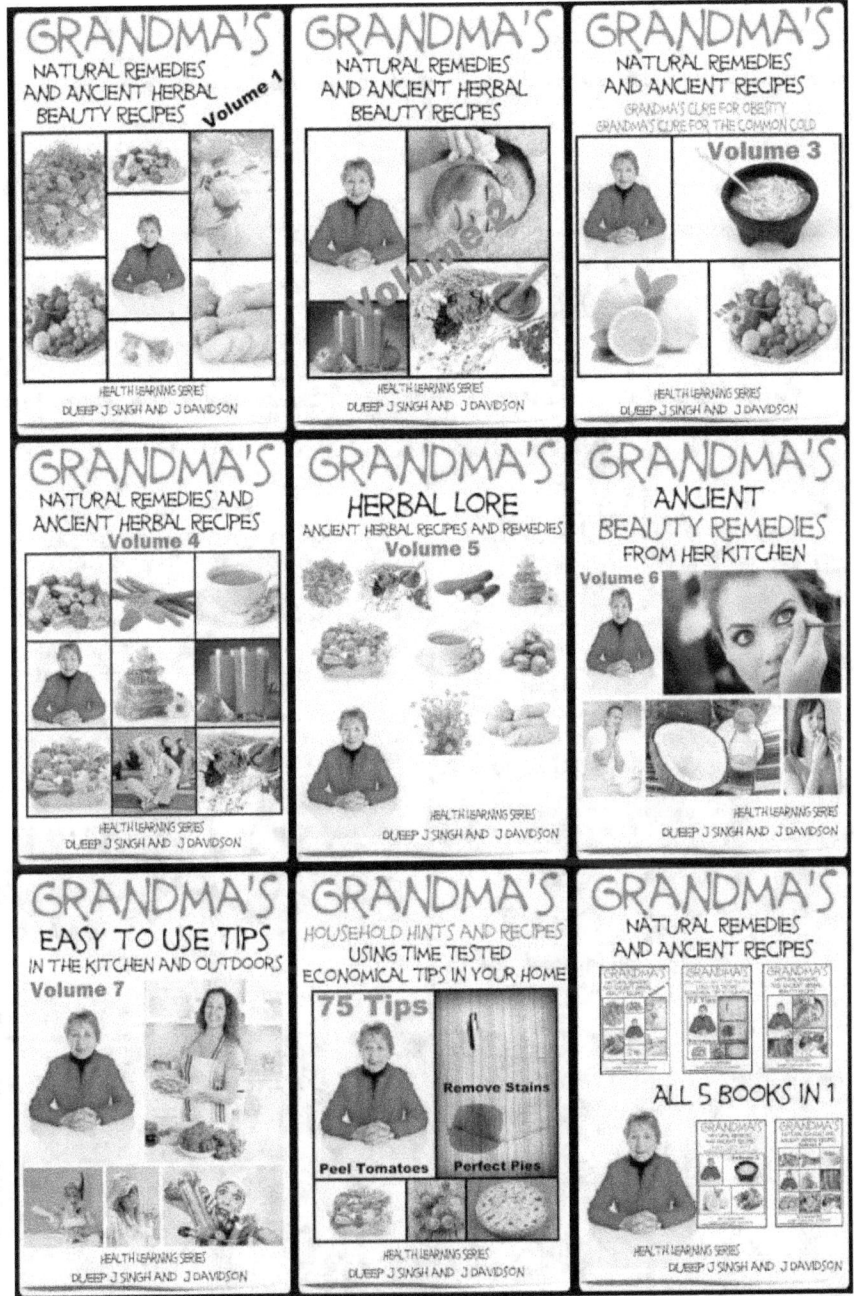

Country Life Books

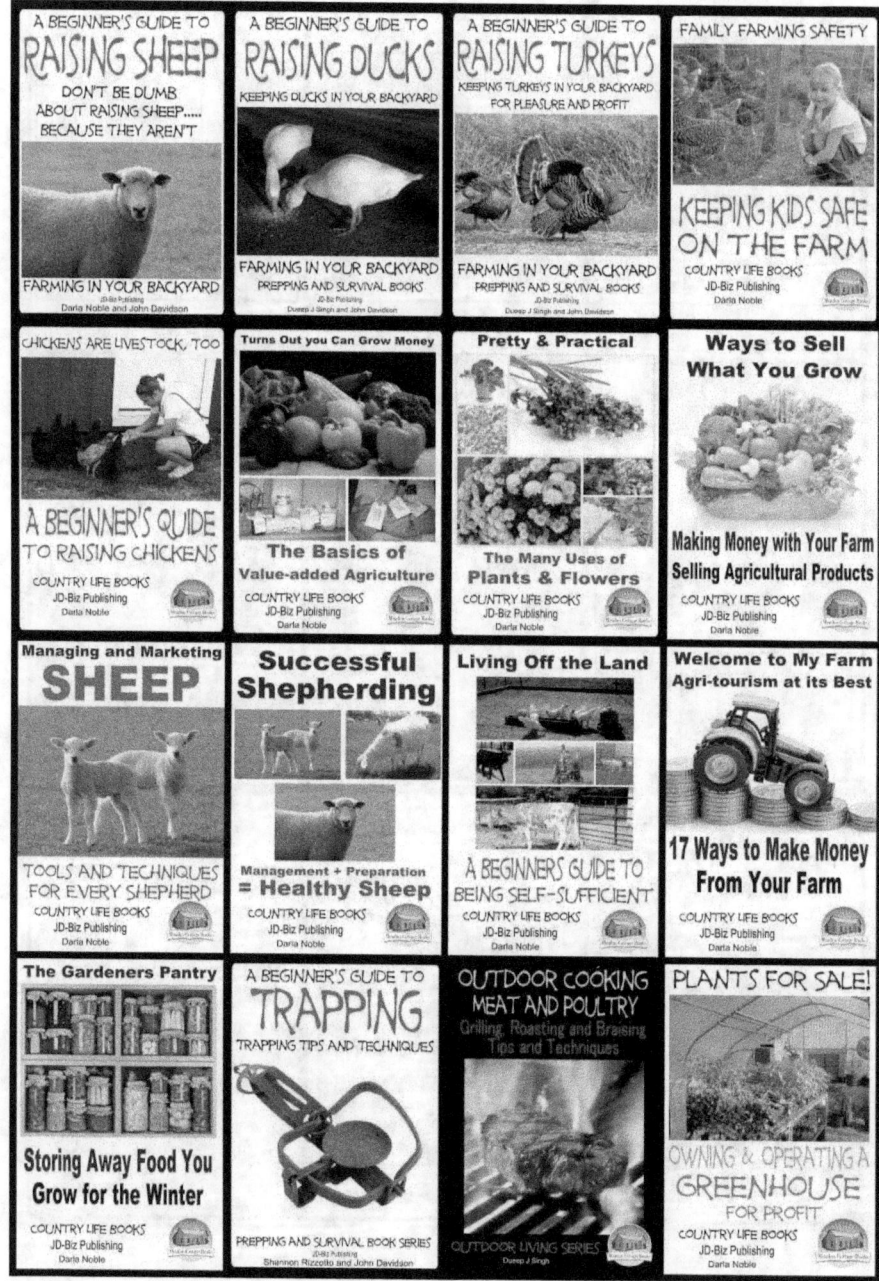

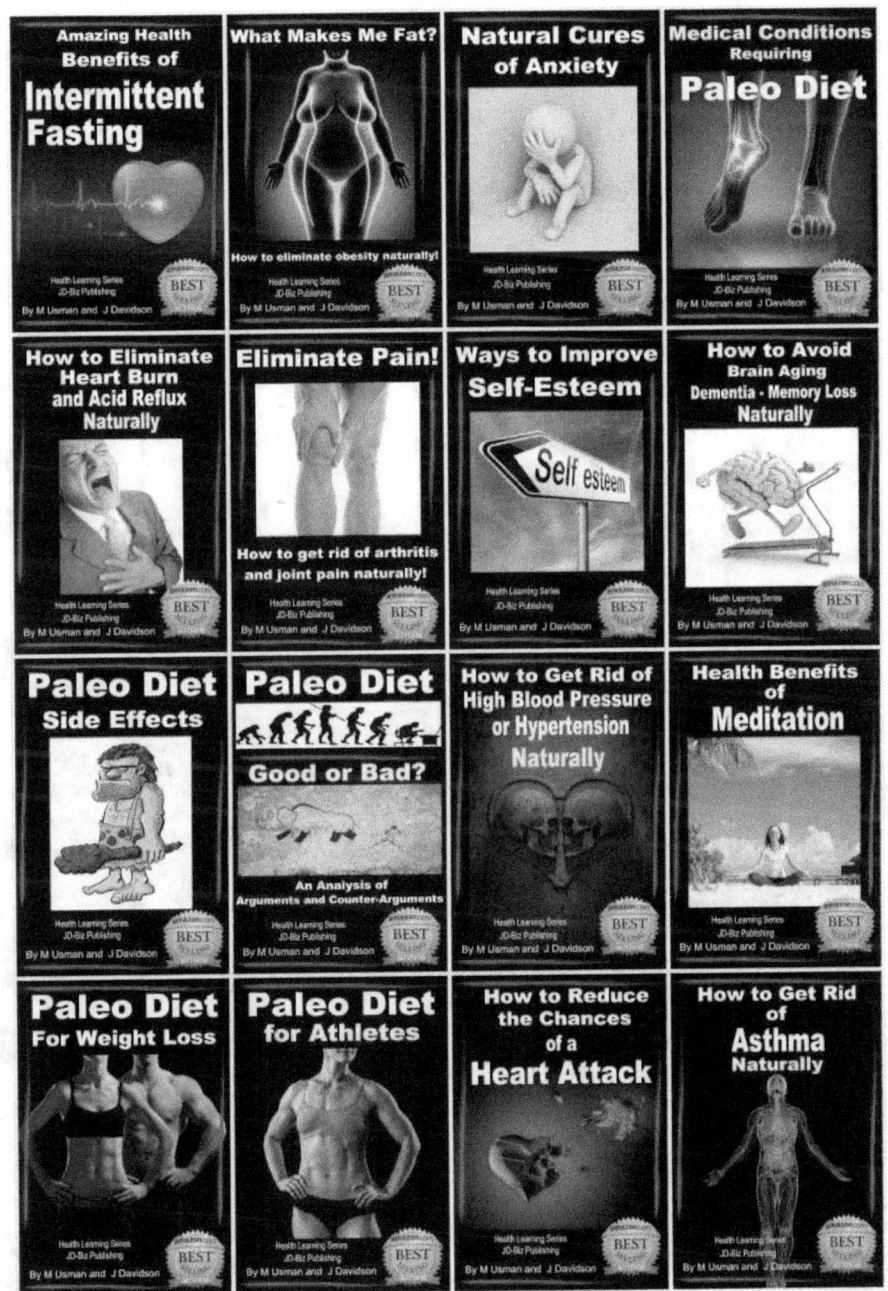

Amazing Animal Book Series

Learn To Draw Series

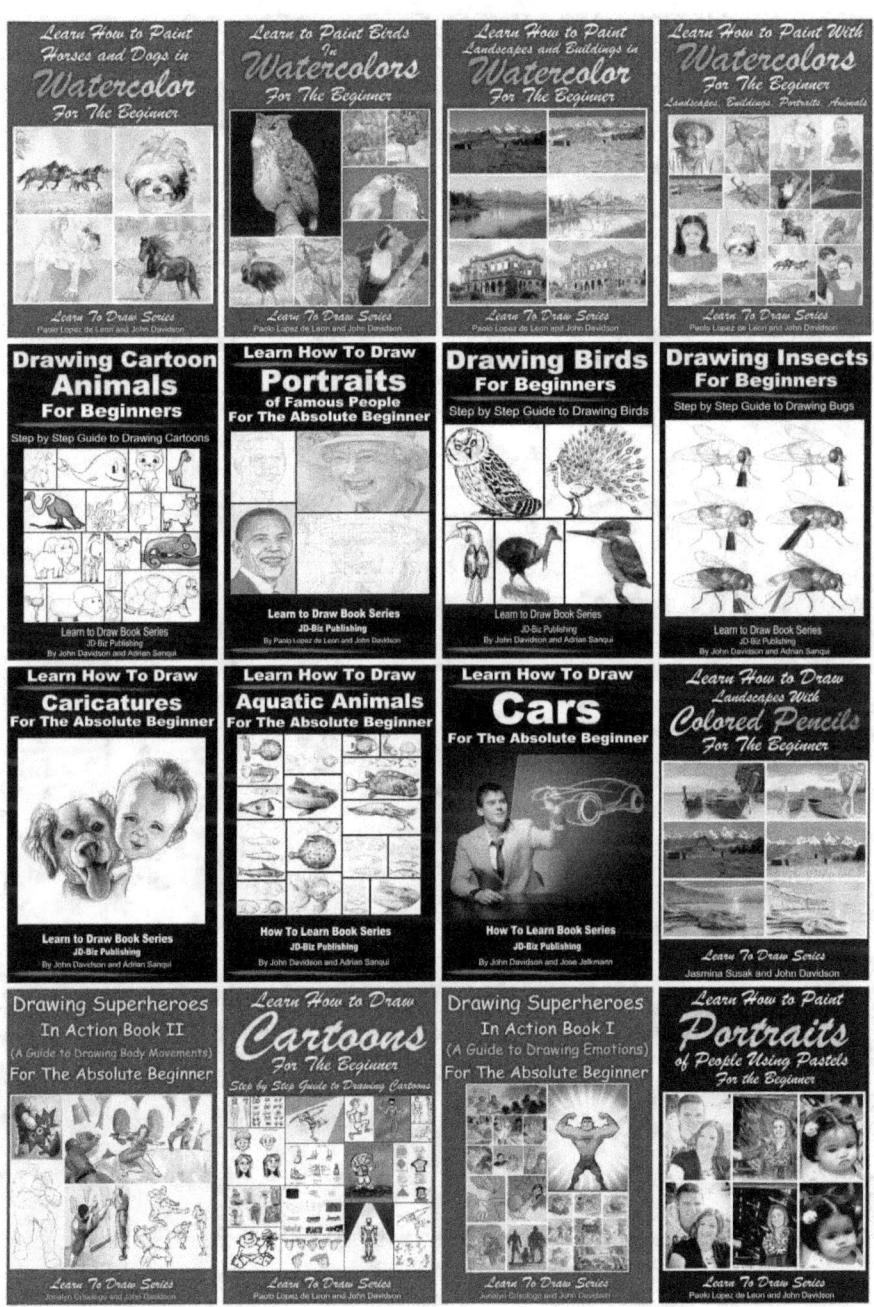

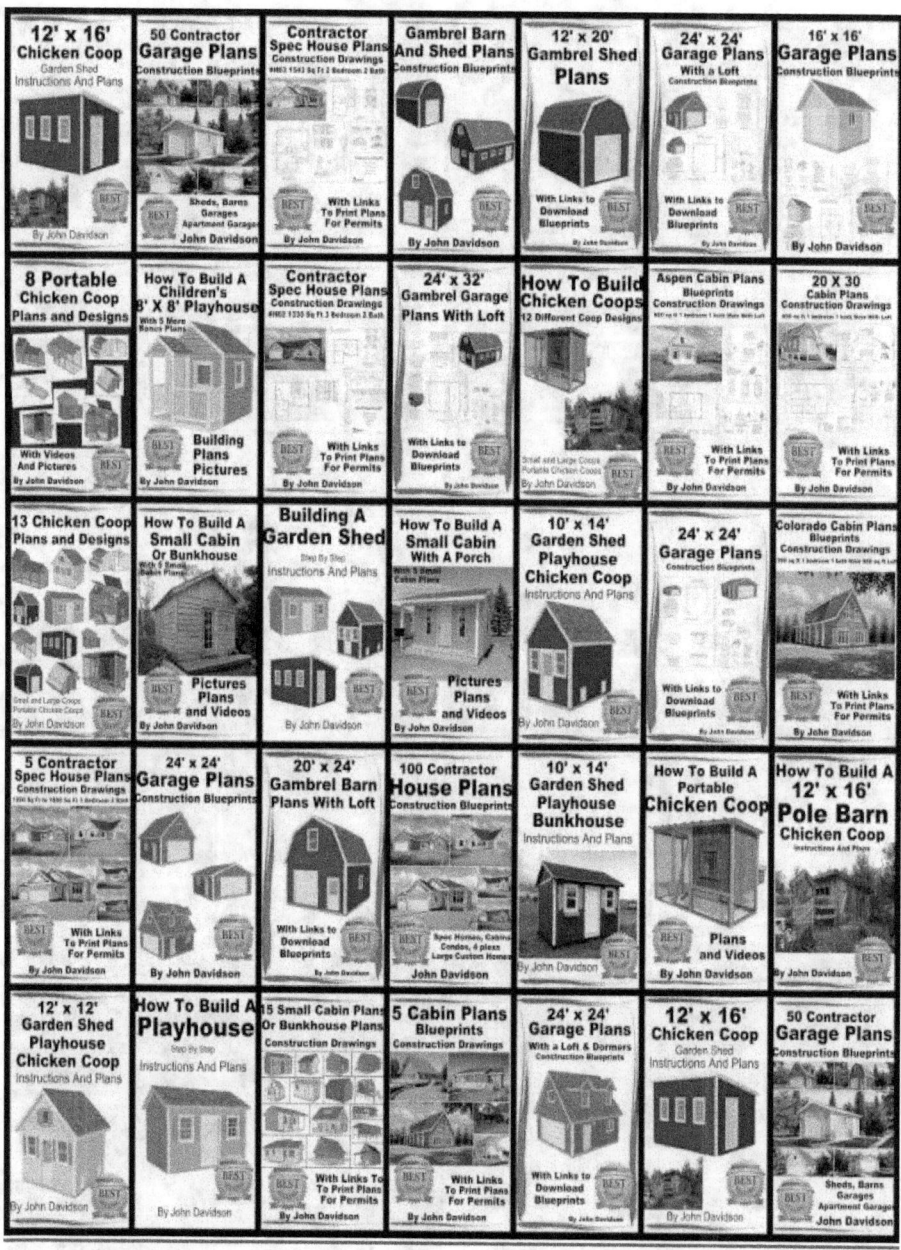

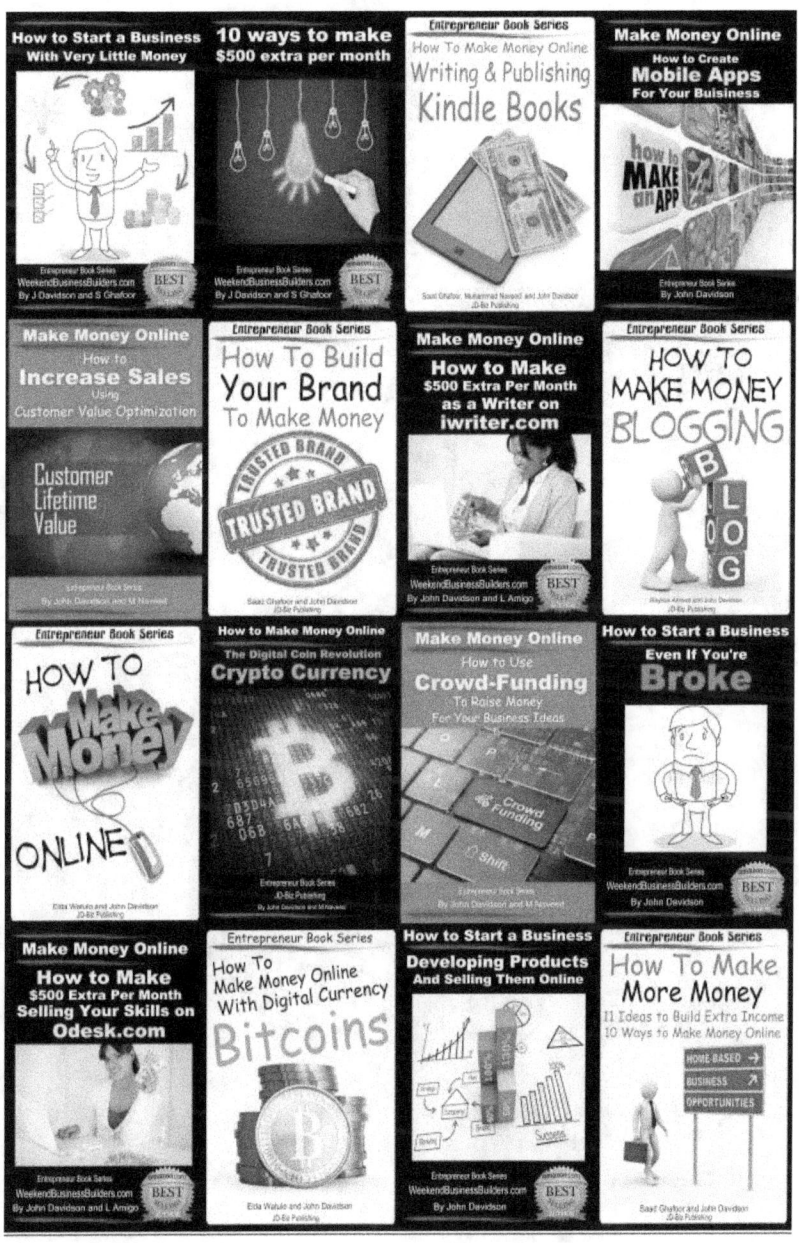

Our books are available at

1. Amazon.com

2. Barnes and Noble

3. Itunes

4. Kobo

5. Smashwords

6. Google Play Books

Publisher

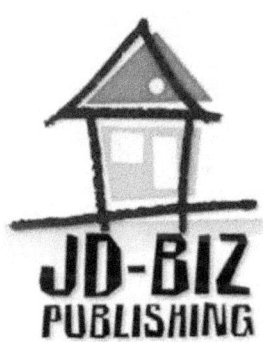

JD-Biz Corp

P O Box 374

Mendon, Utah 84325

http://www.jd-biz.com/

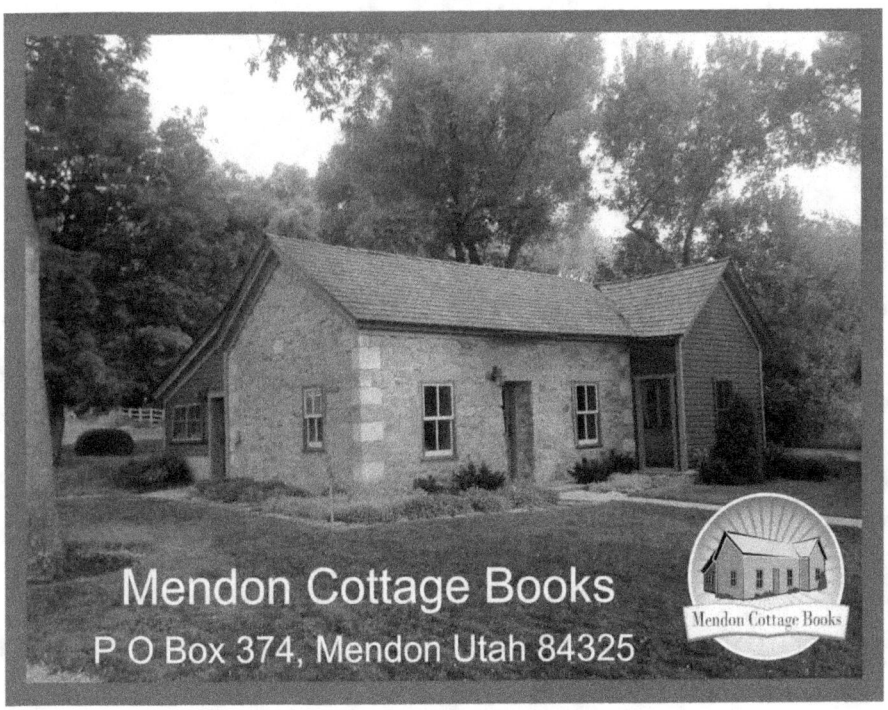

Mendon Cottage Books
P O Box 374, Mendon Utah 84325